Lean and Green Air Fryer Meat Cooking Plan

The Ultimate Lean and Green Meat Recipes for your Air Fryer

Roxana Sutton

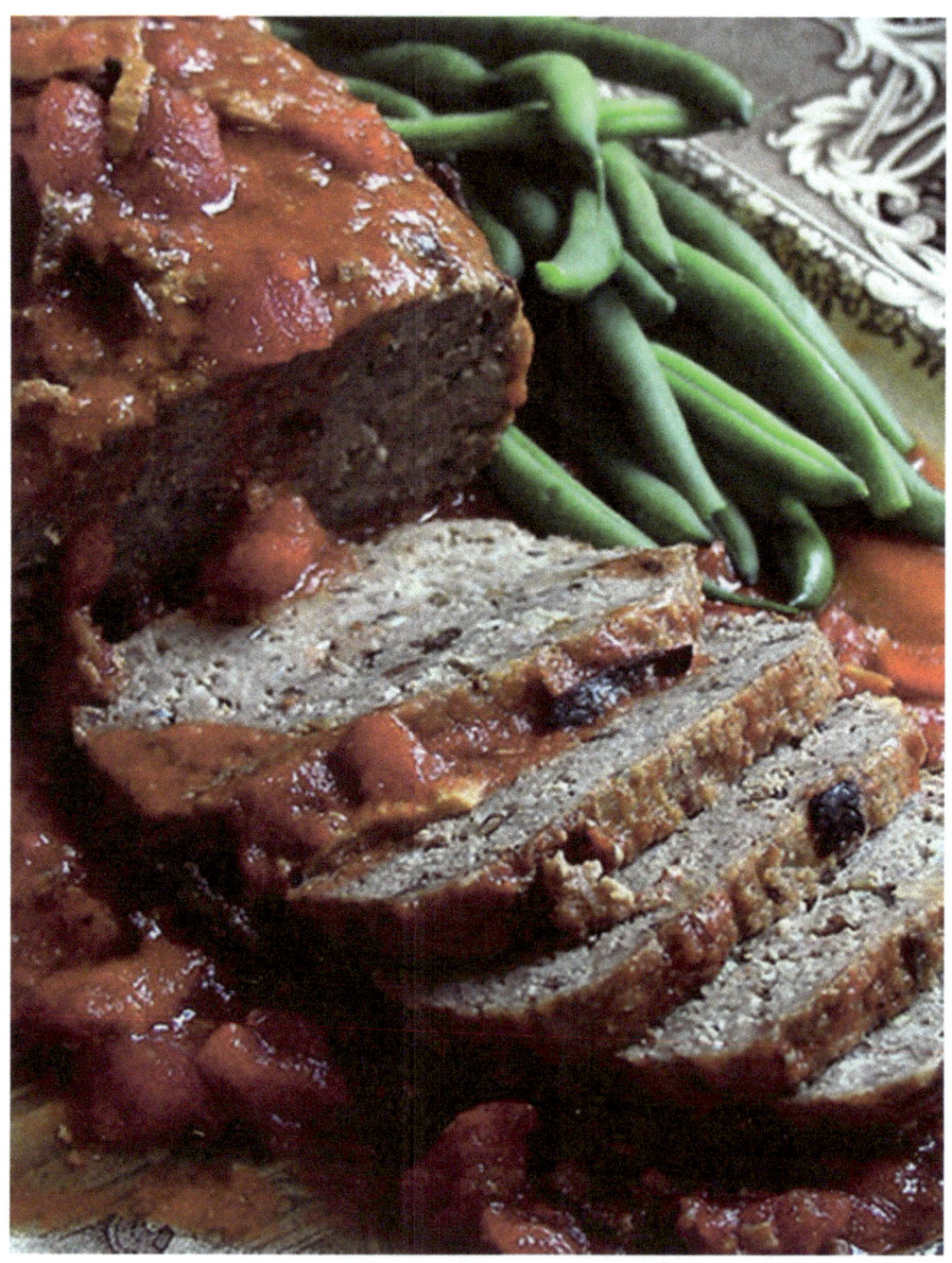

TABLE OF CONTENTS

Leek And Pork Stir Fry

Total Time: 40 mins

Ingredients

- 1 pound pork shoulder thinly sliced (about 500g)
- 2 Tablespoon oyster sauce
- 2 Tablespoon soy sauce
- 1 Tablespoon sesame oil
- 1 teaspoon garlic powder
- 1 teaspoon onion powder
- 1 teaspoon corn starch
- 1/2 teaspoon black pepper
- 1 cup of leek cleaned and sliced diagonally about
- 1/2 inch wide

Instructions

In a large bowl, mix the pork slices with all the seasoning ingredients. Marinate for at least 30 minutes. Lightly grease the inside of the cake barrel.

Put the marinated pork sliced inside the cake barrel. Air fry at 380F (190C) for about 8 minutes, stirring once in the middle

Add the leek to the pork and mix. Air fry again at 380F (190C) for another 4-5 minutes until the pork is cooked through.

Nutrition

Calories: 186kcal | Carbohydrates: 11g | Protein: 16g | Fat: 9g | Saturated Fat: 2g | Cholesterol: 46mg | Sodium: 814mg | Potassium: 370mg | Fiber: 1g | Sugar: 3g | Vitamin C: 8mg | Calcium: 47mg | Iron: 2mg

Hearty Meatball Soup

Prep Time: 10 mins

Cook Time: 45 mins

Ingredients

Meatball Ingredients:

- 1 pound ground meat I used ground turkey, about 500g
- 1/4 cup yellow onion finely chopped
- 1/2 cup Panko breadcrumb
- 1/2 tablespoon Italian seasoning
- 2 tablespoon grated Parmesan cheese
- 1 tablespoon soy sauce
- 2 teaspoon corn starch
- 1 teaspoon garlic powder
- 1 teaspoon onion powder
- 1/4 teaspoon black pepper or to taste

Soup Ingredients:

- 2 tablespoon olive oil
- 1 stalk celery diced
- 2 tablespoon garlic chopped
- 1/4 cup yellow onion diced

- 1/4 cup tomato ketchup
- 1/2 cup carrot diced
- 1   large zucchini diced
- 1/4 cup wine I used rice wine 1 can crushed tomatoes
- 1/2 can corn kernels
- 2   cup broth I used chicken
- 1 tablespoon Italian seasoning
- 2 teaspoon garlic powder
- Salt and pepper to taste

Instructions

Line the fryer basket with a grill mat or a sheet of lightly greased aluminum foil.

In a large bowl, combine all the meatball ingredients. Take about 1 tablespoonful of the mixture and roll it into a ball. Place the meatballs into the fryer basket. Spritz the meatballs with oil and air fry at 380F (190C) for about 8 minutes, shake the basket once in the middle.

In the meantime, pour olive oil into a pot and saute garlic, celery, and onion until fragrant. Add in the rest of the soup ingredient and bring it to boil.

When the meatballs are done, transfer them to the pot. Fill the pot with water just enough to cover all the ingredients. Let it simmer for about 30 minutes.

Serve on its own or with pasta or bread.

Nutrition

Calories: 476kcal | Carbohydrates: 22g | Protein: 24g | Fat: 31g | Saturated Fat: 10g | Cholesterol: 83mg

| Sodium: 1047mg | Potassium: 659mg | Fiber: 3g | Sugar: 8g | Vitamin C: 13mg | Calcium: 112mg | Iron: 4mg

Easy Swedish Meatballs

Prep Time: 15 mins

Cook Time: 25 mins

Ingredients

Ingredients for meatballs:

(makes about 30 meatballs)

- 1 1/2 pound ground meat or ground meat mixtures (about 750g) I used ground turkey
- 1/3 cup Panko breadcrumbs
- 1/2 cup milk
- 1/2 of an onion finely chopped
- 1 large egg
- 2 tablespoon parsley dried or fresh
- 2 tablespoon minced garlic
- 1/3 teaspoon salt
- 1/4 teaspoon black pepper or to taste
- 1/4 teaspoon paprika
- 1/4 teaspoon onion powder

Ingredients For Sauce:

- 1/3 cup butter
- 1/4 cup all-purpose flour
- 2 cups broth I used chicken broth
- 1/2 cup milk
- 1 tablespoon soy sauce
- Salt and pepper to taste

Instructions

Line the fryer basket with a grill mat or a sheet of lightly greased aluminum foil.

In a large bowl, combine all the meatball ingredients and let it rest for 5-10 minutes.

Using the palm of your hands, roll the meat mixture into balls of the desired size. Place them in the fryer basket and air fry at 380F (190C) for 8-12 minutes (depending on the size of the meatballs) until they are cooked through and internal temperature exceeds 165F or 74C)

In the meantime, melt the butter in a wok or a pan. Whisk in flour until it turns brown. Pour in the broth, milk, and soy sauce and bring it to a simmer. Season with salt and pepper to taste. Stir constantly until the sauce thickens.

Serve meatballs and sauce over pasta or mashed potato. Sprinkle some parsley if desired.

Nutrition

Calories: 299kcal | Carbohydrates: 12g | Protein: 31g | Fat: 15g | Saturated Fat: 8g | Cholesterol: 121mg

| Sodium: 723mg | Potassium: 443mg | Fiber: 1g | Sugar: 3g | Vitamin C: 3mg | Calcium: 71mg | Iron: 2mg

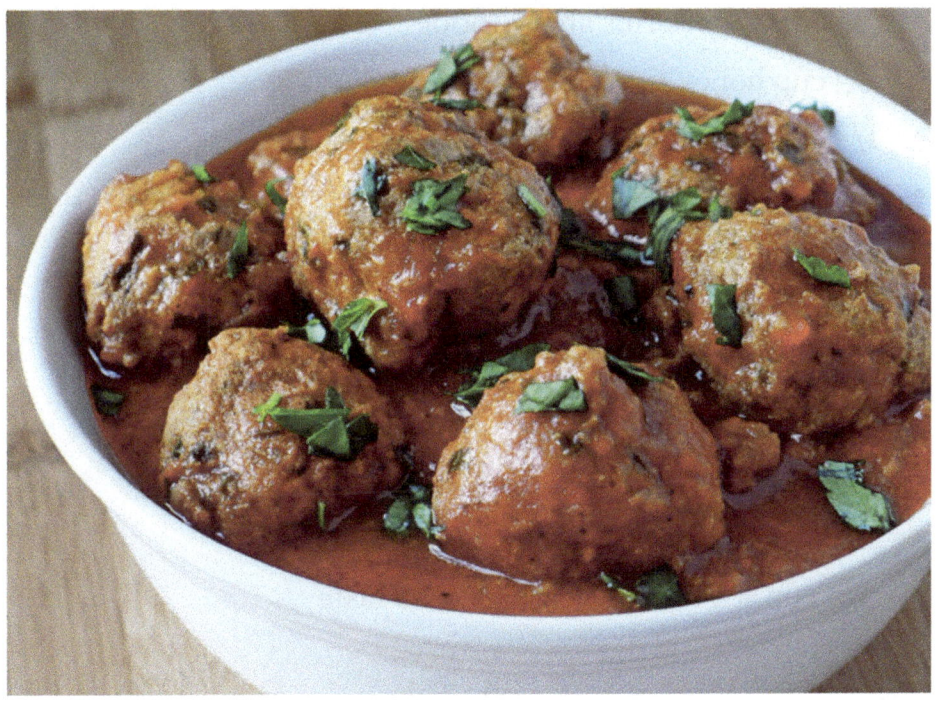

Garlicky Honey Sesame Ribs

Prep Time: 3 hrs

Cook Time: 15 mins

Ingredients

- 2 pounds pork ribs about 1000g
- 1/3 cup honey
- 1/4 cup soy sauce
- 1/4 cup ketchup
- 1/4 cup brown sugar
- 2 tbsp rice vinegar
- 2 tbsp lemon juice
- 2 tsp sesame oil
- 2 Tbsp minced garlic
- 1 Tbsp sesame seeds for garnish or to taste
- 1/4 cup scallions for garnish or to taste

Instructions

In a medium-size bowl, prepare the marinade by mixing honey, soy sauce, ketchup, brown sugar, vinegar, and lemon juice.

Take a Ziploc bag, put the ribs in the bag. Pour about 2/3 of the marinade into the bag, mix with the ribs, and marinate in the refrigerator for at least 3 hours or best overnight. Save the rest of the marinade for later use.

Take the pork ribs out from the refrigerator 30 minutes before air frying.

Line the fryer basket with a grill mat or a sheet of lightly greased aluminum foil.

Put the ribs inside the fryer basket without stacking. Air fry at 380F (190C) for about 10-12 minutes, flip once in the middle until the edges are slightly caramelized.

In the meantime, use a wok to saute garlic in sesame oil until fragrant, about one minute. Then, add in the rest of the marinade. Stir constantly until the sauce thickens.

When the ribs are done, toss the ribs in the wok along with sesame seeds. Sprinkle some scallions on top to serve.

Nutrition

Calories: 429kcal | Carbohydrates: 30g | Protein: 18g | Fat: 27g | Saturated Fat: 8g | Cholesterol: 85mg | Sodium: 721mg | Potassium: 359mg | Fiber: 1g | Sugar: 27g | Vitamin C: 4mg | Calcium: 46mg | Iron: 2mg

Chinese BBQ Pork Pastry

Prep Time: 20 mins

Cook Time: 10 mins

Ingredients

- 1/2 pound char siu Chinese BBQ pork diced (about 250g)
- 2 tsp olive oil
- 1/4 onion diced
- 1 1/2 tbsp ketchup
- 1/2 tbsp oyster sauce
- 1 tbsp sugar
- 1 tbsp honey
- 1/4 cup water
- 1 1/2 tbsp corn starch
- 1 1/2 tbsp water
- 1 roll of store-bought pie crust thawed according to package instruction
- 1 egg beaten

Instructions

In a wok or frying pan, saute diced onion in olive oil until translucent. Then, add in ketchup, oyster sauce, sugar, honey, and 1/4 cup water. Stir and bring to boil

In the meantime, take a small bowl and mix the corn starch with 1 1/2 tablespoon of water. Add the mixture to the wok and stir constantly until the sauce thickens.

Add the diced BBQ pork and stir. Wait for it to cool, then put it in the refrigerator for at least 30 minutes. The refrigeration will cause the mixture to harden and will make it easier to handle later.

Line the fryer basket with a grill mat or lightly greased aluminum foil.

Roll out pie crusts. Use a bowl size of your choice to trace circles onto the pie crust and cut them into circular pieces. Mix the leftover pie crust, use a rolling pin to roll them out. Repeat the above process to get as many circular crusts as you can.

Lay the circular pieces of pie crust on the counter and put the desired amount of BBQ pork filling in the center. Fold pie crust in half and keep the fillings inside. Use the back of a fork to press down on the edges of the pie crust to seal.

Carefully transfer the pork pastry into the fryer basket. Brush the top surface with egg and air fry at 340F (170C) for about 5-6 minutes. Flip the pastries over and brush the top side with egg.

Air fry again at 340F (170C) for another 5-6 minutes until the surface is golden brown.

Nutrition

Calories: 225kcal | Carbohydrates: 17g | Protein: 2g | Fat: 7g | Saturated Fat: 2g | Polyunsaturated Fat: 1g | Monounsaturated Fat: 1g | Trans Fat: 1g | Cholesterol: 100mg | Sodium: 395mg | Potassium: 345mg | Fiber: 1g | Sugar: 17g | Vitamin C: 1mg | Calcium: 8mg | Iron: 1mg

Vietnamese Style Pork Chops

Prep Time: 2 hrs

Cook Time: 10 mins

Ingredients

- 1 pound pork shoulder blade steak (about 500g)
- 3 tbsp dark soy sauce
- 3 tbsp fish sauce
- 2 tbsp minced garlic
- 2 tbsp grated ginger
- 2 tbsp brown sugar
- 1 Lime juice and zest
- 1 tbsp olive oil
- Chopped cilantro to garnish optional

Instructions

Mix the pork with all the pork ingredients, except olive oil and cilantro, and marinate in the refrigerator for at least 2 hours or best overnight. Take the meat out of the refrigerator 30 minutes before air frying. Pat dry the pork steaks with a paper towel. Brush both sides of the meat with olive oil and place them in the fryer basket without stacking. Air fry at 400F (200C) for 8-10 minutes, flip once in the middle until the pork is cooked through when the temperature exceeds 145F or 63C.

Garnish with chopped cilantro if desired.

Nutrition

Calories: 229kcal | Carbohydrates: 23g | Protein: 15g | Fat: 9g | Saturated Fat: 2g | Cholesterol: 46mg | Sodium: 1359mg | Potassium: 322mg | Fiber: 1g | Sugar: 17g | Vitamin C: 7mg | Calcium: 33mg | Iron: 1mg

Meatballs With Gochujang Mayo

Prep Time: 15 mins

Cook Time: 10 mins

Ingredients

Ingredients For Meatballs:

- 1 pound ground pork (about 500g) or meat of your choice
- 1/4 cup onion finely chopped
- 2 Tablespoon soy sauce
- 2 teaspoon corn starch
- 1 teaspoon dried basil
- 1 teaspoon garlic powder
- 1 teaspoon onion powder
- 1/4 teaspoon white pepper powder

Ingredients For Sauce:

- 1 teaspoon Gochujang (Korean hot pepper paste)
- 2 Tablespoon Mayonnaise
- 2Tablespoon mirin

Instructions

Line the fryer basket with a grill mat or a sheet of lightly greased aluminum foil.

Mix all the meatball ingredients then form them into about 1 inch balls. Put the meatballs in the fryer basket without stacking. Spray some oil onto the meatballs and air fry at 380F (190C) for 8-10 minutes until the meat is cooked through at its proper temperature.

In the meantime, take a small bowl and mix all the sauce ingredients. Dip the meatballs in the Gochujang mayo to serve.

Nutrition

Calories: 378kcal | Carbohydrates: 7g | Protein: 21g | Fat: 29g | Saturated Fat: 10g | Cholesterol: 85mg | Sodium: 677mg | Potassium: 368mg | Fiber: 1g | Sugar: 3g | Vitamin C: 2mg | Calcium: 21mg | Iron: 1mg

Five Spices Salt And Pepper Pork

Prep Time: 1 hr 15 mins

Cook Time: 15 mins

Ingredients

Ingredients For Pork:

- 1/2 pound pork shoulder cut into thick slices (about 250g)
- 2 Tablespoon soy sauce
- 1/2 Tablespoon rice wine
- 1 teaspoon corn starch
- 1 Tablespoon minced garlic
- 1 teaspoon sesame oil
- 1/2 teaspoon sugar
- 1/2 teaspoon Chinese five spices powder
- 1/4 cup tapioca starch

Instructions

Marinate the meat with all the pork ingredients, except tapioca flour, for at least 1 hour.

Dredge the pork slices in tapioca flour, shake off excess, and let sit for about 5-10 minutes until you don't see dry flour.

Place the meat in the fryer basket and spray some oil. Air Fry at 380F for 12-14 minutes, flip once in the middle until the surface appears to be nice and crisp.

Toss in the pork slices with chili pepper and chopped cilantro. Then, sprinkle some salt and pepper to serve.

Nutrition

Calories: 100kcal | Carbohydrates: 9g | Protein: 8g | Fat: 3g | Saturated Fat: 1g | Cholesterol: 23mg | Sodium: 529mg | Potassium: 137mg | Fiber: 1g | Sugar: 1g | Vitamin C: 1mg | Calcium: 8mg | Iron: 1mg

Seasoned Pork Chops With Avocado Salsa

Prep Time: 5 mins

Cook Time: 15 mins

Ingredients

- 2 pork chops or pork shoulder blade steaks
- 2 Tablespoon olive oil
- 1 teaspoon sea salt
- 1 teaspoon black pepper
- 1/2 teaspoon paprika
- 1/2 teaspoon garlic powder
- 1/2 teaspoon cumin

Ingredients For Salsa:

- 1 avocado pitted and diced
- 1 large tomato seeded and diced
- 1/3 cup cilantro chopped
- 1 lime juiced
- 1/4 yellow onion finely chopped
- Pickled or fresh jalapeno to taste chopped (optional)

- Salt to taste

Instructions

In a small bowl, mix all the dry seasonings in the pork ingredients and set them aside.

Use a paper towel to pat dry the pork chop then rub both sides with olive oil. Generously season both sides of the meat and air fry at 380F (190C) for 10-12 minutes, flip once in the middle until the internal temperature exceeds 145F (63C).

In the meantime, combine all the ingredients for the salsa in a large bowl.

When the pork chops are done, let them rest for a few minutes. Scoop some salsa over the pork chops to serve.

Nutrition

Calories: 528kcal | Carbohydrates: 18g | Protein: 32g | Fat: 38g | Saturated Fat: 7g | Cholesterol: 90mg | Sodium: 1242mg | Potassium: 1187mg | Fiber: 9g | Sugar: 4g | Vitamin C: 30mg | Calcium: 39mg | Iron: 2mg

Chinese Style Ground Meat Patties

Prep Time: 5 mins

Cook Time: 10 mins

Ingredients

- 1 pound ground pork about 500g
- 1 egg
- 1 teaspoon corn starch
- 1/3 cup green onion chopped
- 1/4 cup cilantro stems chopped
- 1/4 cup yellow onion finely diced
- 2 1/2 Tablespoon oyster sauce
- 2 Tablespoon minced garlic
- 1/4 teaspoon black pepper

Instructions

Mix all the ingredients and making sure everything is well combined.

Line the fryer basket with lightly greased aluminum foil. Form patties of equal size and place them into the fryer basket. Air fry at 380F (190C) for 8-10 minutes until fully cooked when the internal temperature exceeds 160F (72C).

Nutrition

Calories: 335kcal | Carbohydrates: 5g | Protein: 21g | Fat: 25g | Saturated Fat: 9g | Cholesterol: 123mg | Sodium: 390mg | Potassium: 394mg | Fiber: 1g | Sugar: 1g | Vitamin C: 5mg | Calcium: 39mg | Iron: 1mg

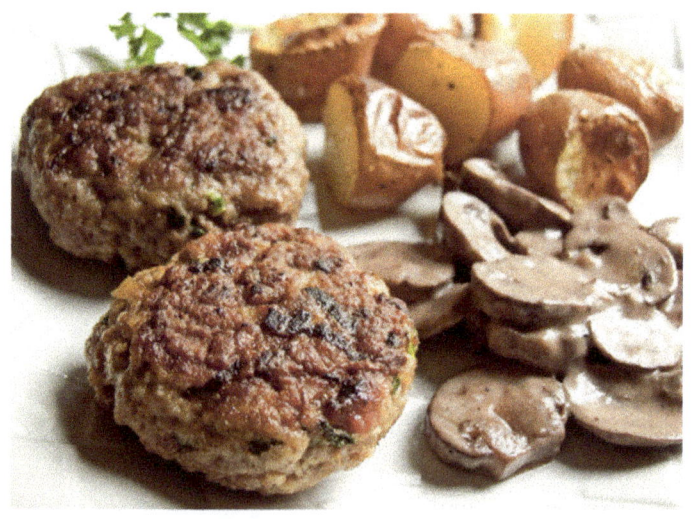

Pork Satay Skewers

Prep Time: 1 hr

Cook Time: 15 mins

Ingredients

Ingredients For Pork:

- 1 pound pork shoulder (about 500g) cut into 1/2 inch cubes
- 1/4 cup soy sauce
- 2 Tablespoons brown sugar
- 2 tablespoons Thai sweet chili sauce
- 1 Tablespoon sesame oil
- 1 Tablespoon minced garlic
- 1 Tablespoon fish sauce

Ingredients For The Sauce:

- 1/3 cup peanut butter
- 3 Tablespoon coconut milk or milk or water
- 2 Tablespoon Thai Sweet Chili Sauce
- 2 teaspoon minced garlic
- 2 teaspoon brown sugar
- 1 teaspoon fish sauce

Instructions

Combine all the ingredients for the pork and marinate for at least 1 hour or overnight.

In the meantime, soak the wooden skewers in water for at least 15 minutes. Also, combine all the ingredients for the dipping sauce and set aside.

Thread the pork cubes onto skewers and place them in the fryer basket. Air fry at 380F (190C) for about 8-10 minutes, flip once in between until the meat is cooked through.

Nutrition

Calories: 363kcal | Carbohydrates: 23g | Protein: 21g | Fat: 22g | Saturated Fat: 7g | Cholesterol: 46mg | Sodium: 1607mg | Potassium: 444mg | Fiber: 1g | Sugar: 18g | Vitamin C: 2mg | Calcium: 33mg | Iron: 2mg

Pork Chop Marinated With Fermented Bean Curd

Prep Time: 2 hrs

Cook Time: 15 mins

Ingredients

Ingredients For Pork:

- 1 pound pork shoulder cut into chunks.
- 1-2 pieces fermented bean curd chunk
- 2 teaspoon rice wine
- 1 Tablespoon dark soy sauce
- 1 Tablespoon brown sugar
- 2 Tablespoon garlic minced

Other ingredients:

- Fried garlic chips to taste
- Thinly sliced green onions to taste

Instructions

Marinate the pork with all the pork ingredients for at least 2 hours or best overnight in the refrigerator. Leave the pork out at room temperature 30 minutes before air frying.

Line the fryer basket with a sheet of lightly greased aluminum foil. Put the pork inside without stacking and air fry at 380F (190C) for about 10-12 minutes until the temperature exceeds 160F (71C).

Sprinkle some fried garlic and green onion to serve.

Nutrition

Calories: 143kcal | Carbohydrates: 9g | Protein: 14g | Fat: 5g | Saturated Fat: 2g | Cholesterol: 46mg | Sodium: 194mg | Potassium: 267mg | Fiber: 1g | Sugar: 6g | Vitamin C: 3mg | Calcium: 20mg | Iron: 1mg

Pork And Bean Curd Strips

Prep Time: 1 hr

Cook Time: 15 mins

Ingredients

Ingredients For Pork:

- 1/2 pound pork shoulder cut into strips (about 250g)
- 2 teaspoon sesame oil
- 2 teaspoon corn starch
- 1 teaspoon sugar
- 1 Tablespoon rice wine

Other ingredients:

- 8 ounces bean curd cut into strips
- 1 teaspoon olive oil
- 4-5 cloves of garlic
- 1/4 cup chicken broth
- 3-4 green onion cut into thin slices
- 1 teaspoon black vinegar optional

Instructions

Marinate the pork strips with all the pork ingredients for at least one hour or overnight.

In the meantime, mix 1 teaspoon of olive oil with bean curd strips. In a lightly greased cake pan, air fry the bean curd at 380F (190C) for 6 minutes, stir once in between. Remove and set aside when done.

Put the garlic on the bottom of the cake pan put pork strips over it. Air fry at 380F (190C) for about 8 minutes, stir once in between.

Add in the chicken broth, bean curd strips, and half of the green onion and mix. Air fry at 380F (190C) for 4-5 minutes until the pork is cooked through.

Mix in the remaining green onion and black vinegar to serve.

Nutrition

Calories: 143kcal | Carbohydrates: 4g | Protein: 12g | Fat: 8g | Saturated Fat: 2g | Cholesterol: 23mg | Sodium: 83mg | Potassium: 142mg | Fiber: 1g | Sugar: 1g | Vitamin C: 2mg | Calcium: 81mg | Iron: 1mg

Marinated Korean Style Pork With Mushroom

Prep Time: 35 mins

Cook Time: 15 mins

Ingredients

Ingredients For The Pork:

- 1/2 pound pork shoulder (about 250g) cut into thin slices
- 1/4 cup Korean BBQ sauce

Other Ingredients:

- 1 Tablespoon garlic minced
- 1/2 cup button mushroom cut into slices
- 1/3 cup carrots sliced
- 1 Tablespoon Korean BBQ sauce
- 1 teaspoon corn starch
- 1/3 cup green onion cut into 1-inch pieces

Instructions

Marinate the pork with Korean BBQ sauce and set aside for 30 minutes.

In a lightly greased cake barrel, put the garlic and carrots on the bottom then put pork slices on top. Air fry at 380F (190C) for about 8-9 minutes, stir once in between.

Mix the rest of the ingredients into the cake pan and air fry again 380F (190C) for 3-4 minutes until pork is cooked through.

Nutrition

Calories: 193kcal | Carbohydrates: 19g | Protein: 17g | Fat: 5g | Saturated Fat: 2g | Cholesterol: 46mg | Sodium: 770mg | Potassium: 426mg | Fiber: 1g | Sugar: 12g | Vitamin C: 7mg | Calcium: 36mg | Iron: 1mg

Cilantro Lime Spiced Pork

Prep Time: 1 hr 10 mins

Cook Time: 15 mins

Ingredient:

- 12 Ounces pork shoulder thinly sliced
- 1 Tablespoon soy sauce
- 1/4 teaspoon cumin
- 1/2 teaspoon curry
- 1/4 teaspoon salt

Other Ingredients:

- 1/4 cup cilantro chopped
- 3-4 Tablespoon of lime juice or to taste

Instructions

Marinate the pork slices with all the ingredients for at least 1 hour.

Line the fryer basket with lightly greased aluminum foil. Place the pork slices in the basket and air fry at 380F (190C) for 10-12 minutes until the pork is cooked through.

When done, mix in cilantro and lime juice to serve.

Nutrition

Calories:162kcal | Carbohydrates: 1g | Protein: 21g | Fat: 8g | Saturated Fat: 3g | Cholesterol: 70mg | Sodium: 874mg |

Potassium: 373mg | Sugar: 1g | Vitamin C: 1mg | Calcium: 15mg | Iron: 2mg

Chinese Style Meatloaf With Pickled Cucumber

Prep Time: 5 mins

Cook Time: 20 mins

Ingredients For Pork:

- 1 pound ground pork about 500g
- 1 egg
- 1/4 cup pickled cucumber chopped
- 1 Tablespoon minced garlic
- 1 Tablespoon soy sauce
- 3 Tablespoon juice from pickled cucumber
- 2 teaspoon of rice wine
- 1 teaspoon sesame oil
- 1 teaspoon sugar
- 2 teaspoon corn starch
- White pepper powder to taste

Other Ingredients:

- Chicken or beef stock
- 1/4 cup thinly sliced scallions to garnish.

Instructions

Mix all the pork ingredients and scoop the meatloaf into each ramekin and put them inside the fryer basket.

Fill the stock up to almost to the rim of the ramekins as the fluid may dry up during the air frying process. Put a sheet of aluminum foil over the ramekins and place a steamer rack on top. Air fry at 360F (170C) for about 15-18 minutes until the meat temperature exceeds 160F (72C).

Sprinkle some green onion on top to serve.

Nutrition

Calories: 336kcal | Carbohydrates: 3g | Protein: 21g | Fat: 26g | Saturated Fat: 9g | Cholesterol: 123mg | Sodium: 331mg | Potassium: 350mg | Sugar: 1g | Vitamin C: 1mg | Calcium: 26mg | Iron: 1mg

Honey Garlic Pork

Prep Time: 35 mins

Cook Time: 15 mins

Ingredients For Pork:

- 1/2 pound pork shoulder thinly sliced
- 1 Tablespoon soy sauce
- 1 teaspoon garlic powder
- 1 teaspoon corn starch
- 1 teaspoon rice wine
- 3 Tablespoon tapioca starch

Ingredients For Sauce:

- 1 Tablespoon sesame oil
- 3 Tablespoon minced garlic
- 2 Tablespoon honey
- 2 Tablespoon Chinese black vinegar
- 1 Tablespoon soy sauce

Instructions

In a Ziploc bag, combine all the ingredients for the pork, except for tapioca starch, and marinate for 30 minutes. Before air frying, add tapioca starch to the bag and shake well. The goal is to have all the pork slices coat with some tapioca starch.

Place a sheet of lightly greased aluminum foil in the fryer basket. Put the pork slices in and try to separate them as much as possible. Air fry at 400F (200C) for about 15 minutes, stir 2-3 times in between until the edges are crispy.

In the meantime, saute garlic with sesame oil in a saucepan for about one minute. Then combine the rest of the ingredients and stir constantly until the sauce thickens.

When the pork is done, toss the pork slices in the sauce to serve.

Nutrition

Calories: 154kcal | Carbohydrates: 17g | Protein: 8g | Fat: 6g | Saturated Fat: 1g | Cholesterol: 23mg | Sodium: 531mg | Potassium: 170mg | Fiber: 1g | Sugar: 9g | Vitamin C: 2mg | Calcium: 16mg | Iron: 1mg

General Tso's Pork

Prep Time: 15 mins

Cook Time: 20 mins

Ingredients For Pork:

- 1 pound pork shoulder cut into slices
- 1 egg beaten
- 2 Tablespoon soy sauce
- 1/4 teaspoon salt
- 1/4 teaspoon black pepper
- 1 teaspoon corn starch
- 1/4 cup tapioca starch

Ingredients for sauce:

- 1 1/2 Tablespoon chili oil
- 2-3 Tablespoon minced garlic
- 1 Tablespoon grated ginger
- 2 Tablespoon soy sauce
- 2 Tablespoon vinegar
- 2 Tablespoon sugar
- 2 teaspoon corn starch mix with 4 teaspoon water

Instructions

In a Ziploc bag, mix all the ingredients for the pork, except tapioca starch, and marinate in the refrigerator for at least one hour. Add the tapioca starch into the bag. Shake the bag or mix gently.

Line the fryer basket with lightly greased aluminum foil. Put the pork slices in and spread them out as much as possible. Air fry at 400F (200C) for 15-17 minutes until the outside is crispy and the meat is cooked through, stir 2-3 times in between.

In the meantime, use a saucepan to saute the garlic and ginger in chili oil for one minute. Add in the rest of the ingredients and bring them to a boil. Add in the corn starch and water mixture, stir until the sauce thickens.

When the pork is done, toss in the sauce to coat. Sprinkle some chopped green onion to serve.

Nutrition

Calories: 235kcal | Carbohydrates: 16g | Protein: 17g | Fat: 11g | Saturated Fat: 3g | Cholesterol: 87mg | Sodium: 1220mg | Potassium: 305mg | Fiber: 1g | Sugar: 6g | Vitamin A: 59IU | Vitamin C: 2mg | Calcium: 23mg | Iron: 2mg

Korean Marinated Pork Belly

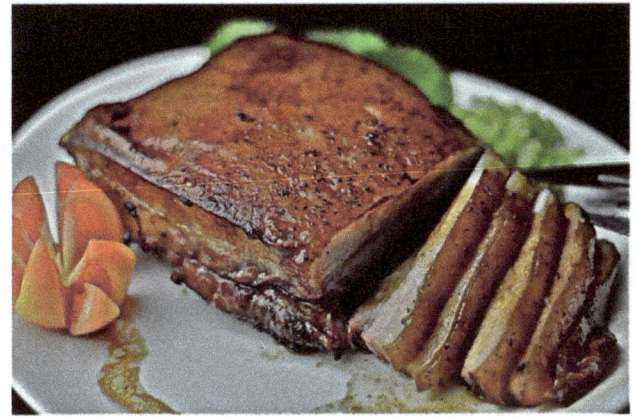

Prep Time: 35 mins

Cook Time: 15 mins

Ingredients

- 1 pound pork belly with or without skin, (about 500g) cut into thin slices
- 2 Tablespoon minced garlic
- 2 Tablespoon minced ginger
- 1/2 tablespoon Korean hot pepper paste Gochujang, or to taste
- 3 tablespoon honey
- 3 tablespoon soy sauce
- 1 tablespoon sesame oil
- 1/2 tablespoon apple cider vinegar

- 3 tablespoon toasted white sesame seeds

Instructions

Prepare the marinade by mixing all other ingredients. Use 3/4 of the marinade to marinate the pork belly for at least 30 minutes and save the rest for later use.

On a lightly greased aluminum foil, air fry the pork belly slices at 380F (190C) for about 12 minutes, stir about 2 times in between, until the meat is cooked through.

In the meantime, use a saucepan to heat the remaining marinade on the stovetop. Stir constantly until the sauce thickens. When the pork is done, toss with the sauce.

To serve, sprinkle some sesame seeds and garnish with cilantro leaves or chopped green onion.

Nutrition

Calories: 360kcal | Carbohydrates: 9g | Protein: 7g | Fat: 33g | Saturated Fat: 11g | Cholesterol: 41mg | Sodium: 397mg | Potassium: 149mg | Fiber: 1g | Sugar: 7g | Vitamin C: 1mg | Calcium: 37mg | Iron: 1mg

Korean Style Pork Chops

Prep Time: 3 hrs

Cook Time: 15 mins

Ingredients

- 1 pound pork chops (about 500g)
- 1/2 cup soy sauce
- 1/3 cup brown sugar
- 1/3 cup onion thinly sliced
- 2 Tablespoon grated ginger
- 2 Tablespoon minced garlic
- 2 teaspoon sesame oil
- 1 teaspoon black pepper
- 1-2 teaspoon Sriracha hot sauce optional
- 3 Tablespoon sliced green onions
- 1 Tablespoon toasted sesame seeds

Instructions

Marinate the pork chops in all the ingredients (except sesame seeds and green onion) in the refrigerator for at least 3 hours.

Take the pork chops out of the refrigerator about 30 minutes before air frying.

Put the pork chops in the parchment paper-lined fryer basket without stacking. Air fry at 380F (190C) for about 15 minutes until the meat temperature is at least 165F (64C).

Sprinkle some green onion and sesame seeds to serve.

Nutrition

Calories: 309kcal | Carbohydrates: 24g | Protein: 28g | Fat: 11g | Saturated Fat: 3g | Cholesterol: 76mg | Sodium: 1709mg | Potassium: 581mg | Fiber: 1g | Sugar: 19g | Vitamin C: 4mg | Calcium: 62mg | Iron: 2mg

Char Siu Pork Chops

Prep Time: 3 hrs

Cook Time: 15 mins

Ingredients

- 1 pound pork chop about 500g
- 1/3 cup of store-bought char siu sauce see notes for substitution
- 2 Tablespoon soy sauce

Instructions

Marinate the pork chops in all the ingredients. Refrigerate for at least 3 hours. Take the pork chops out of the refrigerator 30 minutes before air frying.

Place the pork chops in the parchment paper-lined fryer basket and air fry at 380F (190C) for about 15 minutes until the meat temperature is at least 165F (64C).

Nutrition

Calories: 206kcal | Carbohydrates: 7g | Protein: 25g | Fat: 8g | Saturated Fat: 3g | Polyunsaturated Fat: 1g | Monounsaturated Fat: 1g | Trans Fat: 1g | Cholesterol: 76mg | Sodium: 1032mg | Potassium: 442mg | Fiber: 1g | Sugar: 1g | Calcium: 8mg | Iron: 1mg

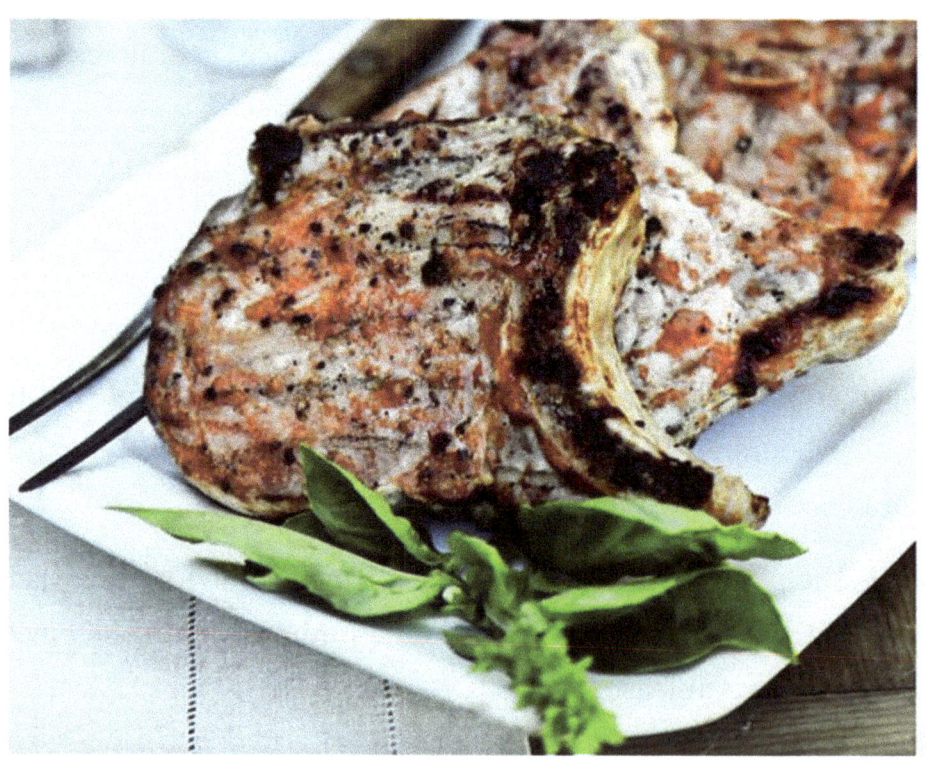

Wasabi Lime Steak

Prep Time: 1 hr 15 mins

Cook Time: 15 mins

Ingredients for the steak:

- 1 pound flank steak (about 500g) thinly sliced
- 1 tablespoon wasabi paste
- 2 Tablespoon soy sauce
- 2 Tablespoon lime juice
- 1/2 Tablespoon Sesame oil
- 1 Tablespoon grated ginger

Wasabi Mayonnaise:

- 1/4 cup mayonnaise
- 1 Tablespoon water
- 1 Tablespoon mirin non-alcohol
- 1 Tablespoon lime juice
- 1 teaspoon wasabi paste

Other ingredients:

- 1/3 cup cilantro chopped

Instructions

Combine all the ingredients for the steak and mix well. Marinate for at least one hour or overnight in the refrigerator.

Line the fryer basket with a sheet of lightly greased aluminum foil. Spread the beef slices out as much as possible and air fry at 380F (190C) for about 8-10 minutes, stir 1-2 times in between.

In the meantime, mix the mayonnaise, water, mirin, lime juice, and wasabi paste in a medium bowl. Drizzle the wasabi mayo over the steak and garnish with some cilantro to serve.

Nutrition

Calories: 288kcal | Carbohydrates: 5g | Protein: 26g | Fat: 18g | Saturated Fat: 4g | Cholesterol: 74mg | Sodium: 686mg | Potassium: 427mg | Fiber: 1g | Sugar: 2g | Vitamin C: 6mg | Calcium: 29mg | Iron: 2mg

Korean Beef With Veggie

Prep Time: 40 mins

Cook Time: 15 mins

Ingredients For Beef:

- 12 ounces flank steak cut into thin slices
- 1 teaspoon corn starch
- 1/4 cup Korean BBQ sauce

Other Ingredients:

- 2 cups mung bean sprouts
- 3 cups baby spinach or spinach cut into 2-inch length
- 1 Tablespoon sesame oil
- 1 Tablespoon minced garlic
- 1 Tablespoon freshly grated ginger
- 1 Tablespoon rice wine
- 2-3 Tablespoon Korean BBQ sauce
- 1 teaspoon jalapeno pepper sliced (optional)
- 1 teaspoon toasted sesame seeds

Instructions

In a large bowl, marinate the beef with Korean BBQ sauce and corn starch for about 30 minutes.

In a small pot, boil the mung bean sprouts until tender. Remove and set aside. Then, boil the spinach for about one minute and set aside.

In a lightly greased cake pan, air fry the marinated beef at 380F (190C) for about 7-8 minutes, stir once in between.

In the meantime, stir fry the garlic, grated ginger, and jalapeno pepper with sesame oil in a wok for about 1-2 minutes until fragrant. Add in the Korean BBQ sauce and rice wine and bring to a boil then turn the stove off.

Toss the spinach, bean sprouts, and beef slices in the sauce. Sprinkle some sesame seeds over the dish to serve.

Nutrition

Calories:220kcal | Carbohydrates: 13g | Protein: 22g | Fat: 8g | Saturated Fat: 2g | Cholesterol: 51mg | Sodium: 486mg | Potassium: 493mg | Fiber: 1g | Sugar: 9g | Vitamin C: 15mg | Calcium: 55mg | Iron: 2mg

Mongolian Beef

Prep Time: 15 mins

Cook Time: 10 mins

Ingredients For The Beef:

- 1 pound flank steak cut into 1/4 inch thick pieces (about 500g)
- 2 teaspoon soy sauce
- 1 teaspoon sesame oil
- 2 teaspoon cornstarch
- 1/4 cup tapioca starch

Ingredients For The Sauce:

- 2 Tablespoon olive oil
- 1 Tablespoon grated ginger
- 1 Tablespoon minced garlic
- 2 Tablespoon soy sauce
- 3 Tablespoon brown sugar
- 3-4 green onion green parts only, cut into 1-2 inch pieces
- 1-2 teaspoon sesame seeds optional

Instructions

In a Ziploc back, marinate the steak pieces with soy sauce, sesame oil, and corn starch for at least 15 minutes. Add in the tapioca starch and shake, making sure all the pieces are coated.

Line the fryer basket with a sheet of lightly greased aluminum foil. Put the steak pieces in, preferably without stacking, and air fry at 400F (200C) for about 8 minutes, flip once until the edges look slightly crispy.

In the meantime, in a frying pan or a wok, saute the garlic and grated ginger in olive oil for about 1-2 minutes until fragrant. Add in the soy sauce and brown sugar and stir constantly until the sauce thickens.

 When the beef is done, toss the beef in the sauce, followed by the green onion. To serve, sprinkle the dish with sesame seeds if desired.

Nutrition

Calories: 306kcal | Carbohydrates: 19g | Protein: 26g | Fat: 14g | Saturated Fat: 4g | Cholesterol: 68mg | Sodium: 735mg | Potassium: 443mg | Fiber: 1g | Sugar: 9g | Vitamin A: 90IU | Vitamin C: 2mg | Calcium: 46mg | Iron: 2mg

Beef Wrapped Cheesy Mushroom

Prep Time: 10 mins

Cook Time: 10 mins

Ingredients

- 12 pieces of thinly sliced beef
- 12 button mushrooms
- 1/3 cup cheddar cheese
- 1/4 cup Korean BBQ sauce
- 2 Tablespoon sesame seeds optional
- 6 pieces of pickled jalapeno peppers chopped (optional)

Instructions

Marinate the beef with Korean BBQ sauce for 15 minutes.

Use a paper towel to wipe the button mushroom clean and remove the stems. Fill the mushroom with cheese and some chopped jalapeno pepper.

Take a slice of beef and wrap it around the mushroom. Air fry at 380F (190C) for about 5 minutes (depending on the thickness of the meat).

Sprinkle some sesame seeds to serve.

Nutrition

Calories: 330kcal | Carbohydrates: 16g | Protein: 29g | Fat: 17g | Saturated Fat: 7g | Cholesterol: 73mg | Sodium: 800mg | Potassium: 718mg | Fiber: 2g | Sugar: 11g | Vitamin C: 3mg | Calcium: 214mg | Iron: 4mg

Cumin Beef

Prep Time: 3 hrs

Cook Time:15 mins

Ingredients

- 1 pound beef flank steak thinly sliced (about 500g)
- 3 Tablespoon Soy sauce
- 2 Tablespoon chopped garlic
- 1 tablespoon Shaoxing wine
- 1 1/2 Tablespoon cumin
- 1 Tablespoon paprika
- 1 1/2 teaspoon corn starch
- 1/4 teaspoon salt
- 1/2 teaspoon black pepper
- 1/2 teaspoon hot pepper flakes optional
- 1/3 cup chopped cilantro
- 1/2 cup chopped green onion

Instructions

Marinate the beef slices with all of the ingredients, except cilantro and green onion, in the refrigerator for at least 3 hours. Remove from the refrigerator about 30 minutes before air frying.

In a lightly greased foiled lined fryer basket, air fry the beef slices at 380F (190C), stir 2-3 times in between, about 10-12 minutes, or until the desired degree of doneness is reached.

When done, toss the beef with cilantro and green onion to serve.

Nutrition

Calories: 196kcal | Carbohydrates: 6g | Protein: 27g | Fat: 6g | Saturated Fat: 2g | Cholesterol: 68mg | Sodium: 968mg | Potassium: 546mg | Fiber: 1g | Sugar: 1g | Vitamin A: 1105IU | Vitamin C: 4mg | Calcium: 68mg | Iron: 4mg

Meatballs With Gochujang Mayo

Prep Time: 15 mins

Cook Time: 10 mins

Ingredients For Meatballs:

- 1 pound ground pork (about 500g) or meat of your choice
- 1/4 cup onion finely chopped
- 2 Tablespoon soy sauce
- 2 teaspoon corn starch
- 1 teaspoon dried basil
- 1 teaspoon garlic powder
- 1 teaspoon onion powder
- 1/4 teaspoon white pepper powder

Ingredients for sauce:

- 1 teaspoon Gochujang (Korean hot pepper paste)
- 2 Tablespoon Mayonnaise
- 2 Tablespoon mirin

Instructions

Line the fryer basket with a grill mat or a sheet of lightly greased aluminum foil.

Mix all the meatball ingredients then form them into about 1 inch balls. Put the meatballs in the fryer basket without stacking. Spray some oil onto the meatballs and air fry at 380F (190C) for 8-10 minutes until the meat is cooked through at its proper temperature.

In the meantime, take a small bowl and mix all the sauce ingredients. Dip the meatballs in the Gochujang mayo to serve.

Nutrition

Calories:378kcal | Carbohydrates: 7g | Protein: 21g | Fat: 29g | Saturated Fat: 10g | Cholesterol: 85mg | Sodium: 677mg | Potassium: 368mg | Fiber: 1g | Sugar: 3g | Vitamin C: 2mg | Calcium: 21mg | Iron: 1mg

Pie Crust Beef Empanadas

Prep Time: 30 mins

Cook Time: 15 mins

Ingredients

- 1 pound ground beef
- 1-2 Tablespoon pickled jalapeno chopped (optional)
- 1 teaspoon corn starch
- 1 teaspoon cumin
- 1 teaspoon chili powder
- 1/4 teaspoon salt or to taste
- 1/4 teaspoon pepper or to taste
- 1 teaspoon olive oil
- 2 Tablespoon minced garlic
- 1/4 cup diced onions
- 2 rolls of pie crust thawed according to package instruction
- 1 cup Mexican blend cheese or to taste
- 1 egg beaten

Instructions

In a large bowl, mix the ground beef with jalapeno (optional), corn starch, cumin, chili powder, salt, and pepper, and let it sit for about 5-10 minutes.

Line the fryer basket with a grill mat or lightly greased aluminum foil.

In a large skillet, saute garlic and onion for about 1 minute until fragrant. Add in the ground beef and stir fry until beef is cooked through and the onion is translucent.

Roll out pie crusts. Use a bowl size of your choice to trace circles onto the piecrust and cut them into circular pieces. Mix the leftover pie crust, use a rolling pin to roll them out. Repeat the above process to get as many circular crusts as you can.

Lay the circular pieces of pie crust on the counter and put the desired amount of filling and cheese in the center. Fold pie crust in half and keep the fillings inside. Use the back of a fork to press down on the edges of the pie crust.

Carefully transfer the empanadas into the fryer basket. Brush the top surface with egg and air fry at 350F (175C) for about 4-5 minutes. Flip the empanadas over and brush the top side with egg. Air fry again at 350F (175C) for another 3-4 minutes until the surface is golden brown.

Nutrition

Calories: 545kcal | Carbohydrates: 30g | Protein: 22g | Fat: 37g | Saturated Fat: 14g | Cholesterol: 99mg

| Sodium: 554mg | Potassium: 318mg | Fiber: 2g | Sugar: 1g | Vitamin C: 1mg | Calcium: 159mg | Iron: 4mg

Tri-tip Roast

Prep Time: 1 hr 10 mins

Cook Time: 30 mins

Ingredients

- 2 pound tri-tip roast excess fat trimmed
- 6-8 garlic cloves
- 1/4 cup olive oil
- 2 1/2 tsp salt
- 1 tsp garlic powder
- 1/2 tsp black pepper

Instructions

In a food processor or a blender, pulse the seasoning ingredient several times. Pat dry the tri-tip roast with a paper towel and put it inside a large Ziploc bag.

Put the seasoning mixture inside the bag, squeeze out as much air as possible and seal the bag. Spread the seasoning and massage the meat at the same time, making sure all surfaces are covered with the mixture. Leave it at room temperature for about one hour.

Insert a meat thermometer into the center of the roast. Air fry at 400F (200C) for about 20-25 minutes until the desired temperature is reached, 125F (52C) for rare, 135F (57C) for medium-rare and 145F (63C) for medium.

Let the roast rest for about 10 minutes before serving.

Nutrition

Calories:323kcal | Carbohydrates: 1g | Protein: 31g | Fat: 21g | Saturated Fat: 6g | Cholesterol: 98mg | Sodium: 1050mg | Potassium: 503mg | Fiber: 1g | Sugar: 1g | Vitamin C: 1mg | Calcium: 42mg | Iron: 2mg

Cheese Stuffed Meatballs

Prep Time: 10 mins

Cook Time: 15 mins

Ingredients

- 1 lb ground beef (about 500g)
- 3/4 cup crushed saltine crackers or breadcrumb
- 1/4 cup onion chopped
- 1/4 cup Parmesan cheese
- 1 tsp onion powder
- 1 tsp garlic powder
- 1 tsp parsley
- 1/2 tsp salt
- 1/4 tsp pepper
- 2 eggs
- 3 sticks mozzarella cheese cut into 4-5 pieces each

Other Ingredients:

- Spaghetti sauce

Instructions

Line the fryer basket with a grill mat or lightly greased aluminum foil.

Mix all the ingredients, except mozzarella cheese. Scoop about 2 Tablespoons of the meat mixture and wrap one piece of the cheese in the middle to form a ball. Place the meatballs inside the air fryer.

Spray the meatballs with some oil. Air fry at 380F (190C) for about 6 minutes. Flip, spray some oil again, and air fry at 380F (190C) for another 4-5 minutes.

Take a pot to heat the spaghetti sauce. When the meatballs are done, simmer the meatballs in the sauce for a few minutes.

Serve the meatballs and sauce with your favorite pasta.

Nutrition

Calories: 312kcal | Carbohydrates: 9g | Protein: 20g | Fat: 21g | Saturated Fat: 9g | Cholesterol: 119mg | Sodium: 532mg | Potassium: 254mg | Fiber: 1g | Sugar: 1g | Vitamin A: 112IU | Vitamin C: 1mg | Calcium: 83mg | Iron: 2mg

Asian Meatball Stuffed Zucchini

Prep Time: 15 mins

Cook Time: 15 mins

Ingredients

- 1 pound ground beef (about 500g)
- 1 egg beaten
- 1/4 cup minced onion
- 2 tbsp chopped basil
- 2 tbsp oyster sauce
- 1 tsp corn starch
- 1/4 tsp black pepper or to taste
- 2 large zucchinis peeled

Instructions

Combine all the ingredients, except zucchini, and let it marinate at room temperature for about 15 minutes.

Line the fryer basket with a large sheet of aluminum and spray it with some oil.

Cut zucchini into 1-inch sections and hollow out the center with a sharp knife. Then, fill the zucchini with the beef mixture and put them into the fryer basket without stacking.

Air fry at 360F (180C) for 10-12 minutes. Flip sides about halfway through and continue to air fry until the ground meat is cooked through when then internal temperature exceeds 160F (72C).

Nutrition

Calories: 221kcal | Carbohydrates: 4g | Protein: 15g | Fat: 16g | Saturated Fat: 6g | Cholesterol: 81mg | Sodium: 231mg | Potassium: 394mg | Fiber: 1g | Sugar: 2g | Vitamin C: 12mg | Calcium: 30mg | Iron: 2mg

Air Fried Bulgogi

Prep Time: 30 mins

Cook Time: 10 mins

Ingredients

- 1 pound thinly sliced beef rib-eye
- 1/4 cup thinly sliced onion
- 1/3 cup Korean BBQ Sauce or to taste
- 2 tbsp grated ginger
- 1/4 cup thinly sliced green onion
- 2 tsp sesame seed

Instructions

In a large Ziploc bag, combine the meat, onion, Korean BBQ sauce, and ginger and mix well. Marinate for at least 30 minutes.

Lin the fryer basket with a grill mat or a sheet of lightly greased aluminum foil.

Spread the beef out inside the basket as much as possible and air fry at 380F (190C) for 8-10 minutes, stir once in the middle until the meat is cooked through.

Sprinkle with sesame seeds and green onion to serve.

Nutrition

Calories: 283kcal | Carbohydrates: 9g | Protein: 24g | Fat: 17g | Saturated Fat: 7g | Cholesterol: 69mg | Sodium: 433mg | Potassium: 361mg | Fiber: 1g | Sugar: 6g | Vitamin C: 2mg | Calcium: 22mg | Iron: 2mg

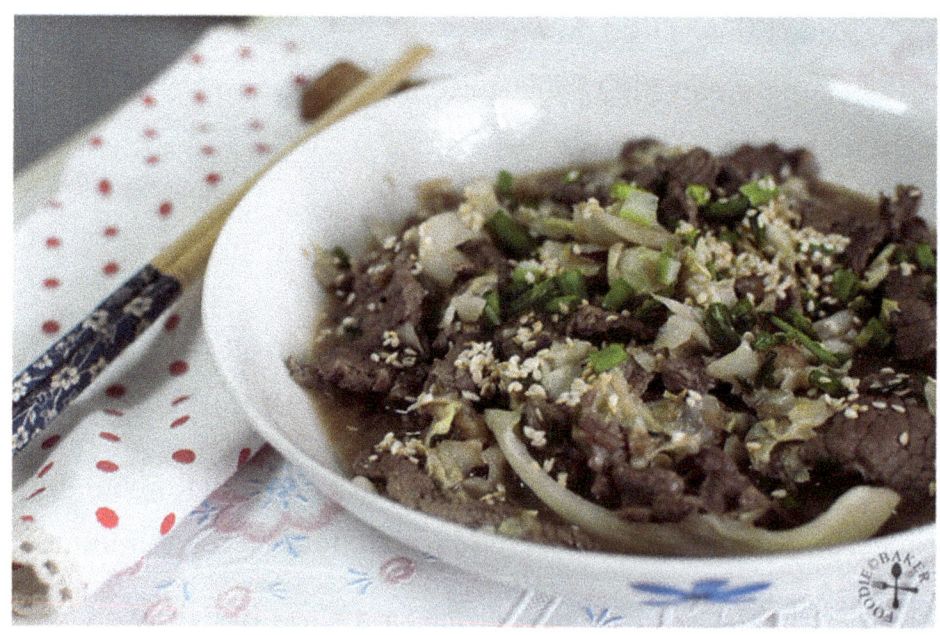

Black Pepper Steak And Mushroom

Prep Time: 1 hr 15 mins

Cook Time: 15 mins

Ingredients For Steak:

- 1 pound rib eye steak about 500g, cubed (about 1/2 inch pieces)
- 1 tsp cornstarch
- 1ntbsp rice wine
- 1 tbsp lime juice
- 2 tsp light soy sauce
- 2 tsp dark soy sauce
- 2 tbsp grated ginger
- 1/4 tsp black pepper or to taste

Other Ingredients:

- 8 button mushrooms thinly sliced
- 1 tbsp garlic finely chopped
- 1 tbsp oyster sauce

Instructions

In a Ziploc bag, mix all the ingredients for the steak and marinate for about one hour. Line the fryer basket with a sheet of lightly greased aluminum foil.

Put the steak inside the fryer basket and air fry at 380F (190C) for about 5 minutes.

Add all other ingredients to the steak and stir. Air fry at 380F (190C) for another 4-5 minutes or until the desired doneness is reached.

Carefully pour the drippings from aluminum foil into a wok and bring it to a boil. Stir constantly until the sauce thickens.

Toss the steak cubes in the wok to coat. Serve immediately.

Nutrition

Calories:275kcal | Carbohydrates: 7g | Protein: 25g | Fat: 16g | Saturated Fat: 7g | Cholesterol: 69mg | Sodium: 407mg | Potassium: 446mg | Fiber: 1g | Sugar: 3g | Vitamin C: 3mg | Calcium: 12mg | Iron: 2mg

Marinated Rib-Eye Steak

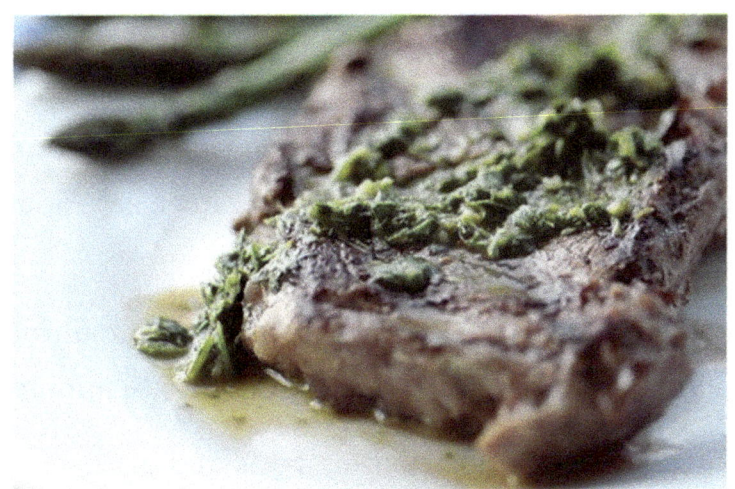

Prep Time: 2 hrs

Cook Time: 10 mins

Ingredients

- 1 pound rib-eye steak (or any cut you prefer) 500g
- 2 Tablespoon grated Ginger
- 2 Tablespoon Honey
- 1 Tablespoon minced garlic
- 1 Tablespoon sesame oil
- 2 teaspoon apple cider vinegar
- 1/4 cup soy sauce

- 1 teaspoon scallion optional
- 1 teaspoon dried minced garlic optional

Instructions

Combine all the seasoning ingredients, except scallions and fried minced garlic, and marinate the steak in a Ziploc bag for at least 2 hours or best overnight in the refrigerator.

If refrigerated, remove from the fridge about 30 minutes before air frying. Preheat air fryer for 400F (200C) for 3-4 minutes.

Place the steak in the preheated air fryer and air fry at 400F (200C) for 6-8 minutes, flip once in the middle, until the desired doneness is reached.

Let the steak rest for about 10 minutes before cutting. Sprinkle some fried minced garlic and scallions to serve if desired.

Nutrition

Calories: 317kcal | Carbohydrates: 11g | Protein: 25g | Fat: 20g | Saturated Fat: 8g | Cholesterol: 69mg | Sodium: 870mg | Potassium: 349mg | Fiber: 1g | Sugar: 9g | Vitamin C: 1mg | Calcium: 19mg | Iron: 2mg

Asian Flavored Ribs

Prep Time: 2 hrs 15 mins

Cook Time: 10 mins

Ingredients

- 1 pound beef short ribs about 500g
- 1/3 cup brown sugar
- 1/4 cup oyster sauce
- 1/4 cup soy sauce
- 2 tbsp rice wine
- 3 cloves garlic minced
- 1 tbsp fresh grated ginger
- 1 tbsp scallions

Instructions

Put the short ribs in a large Ziploc bag.

In a large bowl, mix all other ingredients, except scallions. Pour the mixture into the Ziploc bag and mix it with the ribs. Marinate the ribs for about 2 hours.

Line the fryer basket with a sheet of lightly greased aluminum foil.

Place the ribs inside the fryer basket, without stacking. Air fry at 380F (190C) for 8-10 minutes, flip once in the middle until the surface is slightly caramelized.

Sprinkle some scallions to garnish.

Nutrition

Calories: 244kcal | Carbohydrates: 22g | Protein: 18g | Fat: 9g | Saturated Fat: 4g | Cholesterol: 49mg | Sodium: 867mg | Potassium: 360mg | Fiber: 1g | Sugar: 18g | Vitamin C: 1mg | Calcium: 33mg | Iron: 2mg

Korean Ground Beef Stir Fry

Prep Time: 5 mins

Cook Time: 10 mins

Ingredients

- 1/2 pound ground beef (or ground meat of your choice) about 500g
- 1 teaspoon corn starch
- 1/4 cup Korean BBQ sauce (**see note) or to taste
- 1/4 cup zucchini julienned
- 1/4 cup steamed carrots julienned
- 1 tablespoon sesame seeds
- 1/4 cup scallions

Instructions

In a large bowl, mix the ground beef, corn starch, and Korean BBQ sauce. Marinate for about 5 minutes.

Add the carrots and zucchini to the bowl, and gently mix.

Transfer the mixture to a lightly greased cake barrel and use a spatula to spread them out a bit. Air fry at 380F (190C) for 8-10 minutes, stirring twice in the middle until the ground beef is cooked through. Sprinkle some sesame seeds and scallions to serve.

Nutrition

Calories: 189kcal | Carbohydrates: 7g | Protein: 11g | Fat: 12g | Saturated Fat: 5g | Cholesterol: 40mg | Sodium: 325mg | Potassium: 226mg | Fiber: 1g | Sugar: 5g | Vitamin C: 3mg | Calcium: 37mg | Iron: 1mg

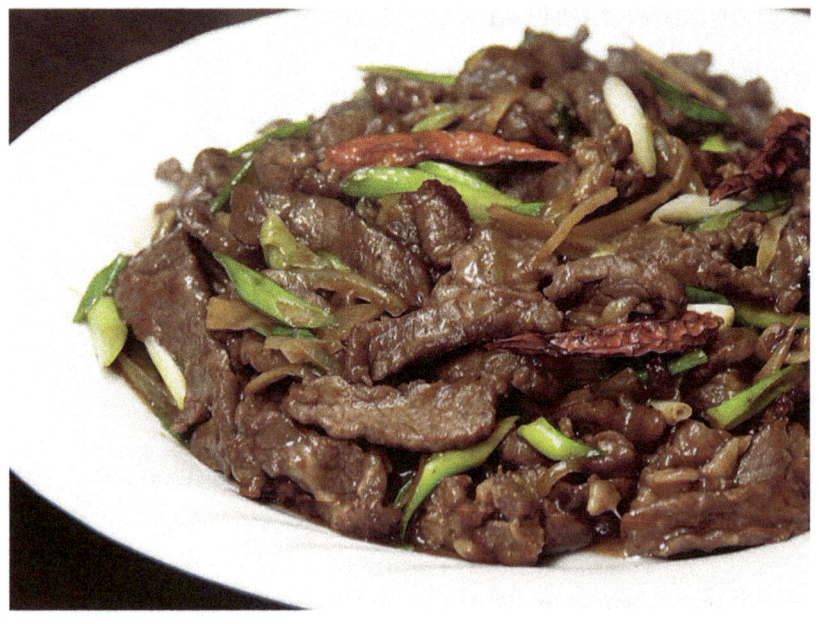

Easy Swedish Meatballs

Prep Time: 15 mins

Cook Time: 25 mins

Ingredients For Meatballs: (Makes About 30 Meatballs)

- 1 1/2 pound ground meat or ground meat mixtures (about 750g) I used ground turkey
- 1/3 cup Panko breadcrumbs
- 1/2 cup milk
- 1/2 of an onion finely chopped
- 1 large egg
- 2 tablespoon parsley dried or fresh
- 2 tablespoon minced garlic
- 1/3 teaspoon salt
- 1/4 teaspoon black pepper or to taste
- 1/4 teaspoon paprika
- 1/4 teaspoon onion powder

Ingredients For Sauce:

- 1/3 cup butter
- 1/4 cup all-purpose flour
- 2 cups broth I used chicken broth

- 1/2 cup milk
- 1 tablespoon soy sauce
- Salt and pepper to taste

Instructions

Line the fryer basket with a grill mat or a sheet of lightly greased aluminum foil.

In a large bowl, combine all the meatball ingredients and let it rest for 5-10 minutes.

Using the palm of your hands, roll the meat mixture into balls of the desired size. Place them in the fryer basket and air fry at 380F (190C) for 8-12 minutes (depending on the size of the meatballs) until they are cooked through and internal temperature exceeds 165F or 74C)

In the meantime, melt the butter in a wok or a pan. Whisk in flour until it turns brown. Pour in the broth, milk, and soy sauce and bring it to a simmer. Season with salt and pepper to taste. Stir constantly until the sauce thickens.

Serve meatballs and sauce over pasta or mashed potato. Sprinkle some parsley if desired.

Nutrition

Calories: 299kcal | Carbohydrates: 12g | Protein: 31g | Fat: 15g | Saturated Fat: 8g | Cholesterol: 121mg

| Sodium: 723mg | Potassium: 443mg | Fiber: 1g | Sugar: 3g | Vitamin C: 3mg | Calcium: 71mg | Iron: 2mg

Korean Kimchi Beef

Prep Time: 30 mins

Cook Time: 10 mins

Ingredients For Beef:

- 1 pound tri-tip strip about 500g, thinly sliced
- 1/4 cup kimchi juice
- 1 tablespoon oyster sauce
- 1 tablespoon soy sauce
- 1 tablespoon freshly grated ginger
- 1 teaspoon sesame oil
- 1 teaspoon corn starch

Other Ingredients:

- 1/2 cup kimchi or to taste
- 1/4 cup thinly sliced green onion
- 1 teaspoon sesame seeds optional

Instructions

In a large bowl, combine all the beef ingredients and marinate for at least 30 minutes.

Line the fryer basket with a sheet of lightly greased aluminum foil.

Transfer the content of the bowl to the fryer basket and air fry at 380F (190C) for 5 minutes. Stir once in the middle.

Add the kimchi and green onion to the beef and stir. Air fry again at 380F (190C) for about 3 minutes. Sprinkle some toasted sesame seeds to serve if desired.

Nutrition

Calories: 200kcal | Carbohydrates: 2g | Protein: 24g | Fat: 10g | Saturated Fat: 3g | Cholesterol: 74mg | Sodium: 436mg | Potassium: 391mg | Fiber: 1g | Sugar: 1g | Vitamin C: 1mg | Calcium: 37mg | Iron: 2mg

A Minnesotan's Beef And Macaroni Hotdish

Prep: 15 mins

Cook: 25 mins

Total: 40 mins

Ingredient

- 1 pound ground beef
- 2 cups elbow macaroni
- ½ large green bell pepper, coarsely chopped
- ½ large onion, chopped
- 1 (16 ounces) can tomato sauce
- 1 pound tomatoes, coarsely chopped
- 2 teaspoons Worcestershire sauce
- 1 teaspoon soy sauce
- 1 teaspoon salt
- ¾ teaspoon dried basil
- ¾ teaspoon dried oregano
- ½ teaspoon ground black pepper
- ½ teaspoon chili powder
- ¼ teaspoon garlic powder

- ⅛ teaspoon hot pepper sauce (such as Tabasco®)
- 1 cup beef broth

Instructions

Cook beef in a large skillet over medium heat, stirring occasionally, until browned, about 5 minutes. Transfer beef to a bowl.

Cook macaroni, bell pepper, and onion in the same skillet over medium heat for 3 minutes. Add cooked beef, tomato sauce, tomatoes, Worcestershire sauce, soy sauce, salt, basil, oregano, ground black pepper, chili powder, garlic powder, and hot pepper sauce. Pour in beef broth. Cover skillet and simmer until macaroni is tender about 15 minutes. Remove lid and simmer, stirring occasionally, until thickened, 5 to 10 minutes.

Nutrition Facts

Calories:336| Protein:19.6g| Carbohydrates:35.9g| Fat:12.8g| Cholesterol: 46.4mg| Sodium: 1039.5mg.

Tennessee Meatloaf

Prep Time: 40 mins

Cook Time: 1 hr

Additional Time: 15 mins

Total Time: 1 hr 55 mins

Ingredients

Brown Sugar Glaze:

- ½ cup ketchup
- ¼ cup brown sugar
- 2 tablespoons cider vinegar

Meatloaf:

- Cooking spray
- 1 onion, chopped
- ½ green bell pepper, chopped
- 2 cloves garlic, minced
- 2 large eggs, lightly beaten
- 1 teaspoon dried thyme
- 1 teaspoon seasoned salt
- ½ teaspoon ground black pepper

- 2 teaspoons prepared mustard
- 2 teaspoons worcestershire sauce
- ½ teaspoon hot pepper sauce (such as tabasco®)
- ½ cup milk
- ⅔ cup Quick-cooking oats
- 1 pound ground beef
- ½ pound ground pork
- ½ pound ground veal

Instructions

Combine ketchup, brown sugar, and cider vinegar in a bowl; mix well.

Preheat oven to 350 degrees F (175 degrees C). Spray two 9x5-inch loaf pans with cooking spray or line with aluminum foil for easier cleanup (see Cook's Note).

Place onion and green pepper in a covered microwave container and cook until softened, 1 to 2 minutes. Set aside to cool.

In a large mixing bowl, combine garlic, eggs, thyme, seasoned salt, black pepper, mustard, Worcestershire sauce, hot sauce, milk, and oats. Mix well. Stir in cooked onion and green pepper. Add ground beef, pork, and veal. With gloved hands, work all ingredients together until completely mixed and uniform.

Divide meatloaf mixture in half and pat half of mixture into each prepared loaf pan. Brush loaves with half of the glaze; set the remainder of glaze aside.

Bake in preheated oven for 50 minutes. Remove pans from oven; carefully drain fat. Brush loaves with remaining glaze. Return to oven and bake for 10 minutes more. Remove pans from the oven and allow the meatloaf to stand for 15 minutes before slicing.

Nutrition Facts

Calories: 233| Protein: 17.1g| Carbohydrates: 15.9g| Fat: 11.2g|Cholesterol: 92mg| Sodium: 324.1mg.

Peruvian Roast Chicken With Green Sauce

Prep Time: 8 hrs

Cook Time: 20 mins

Ingredient

For The Chicken

- 4 pieces of skin-on chicken thighs
- 3 tablespoon olive oil
- 1/4 cup lime juice
- 4 garlic cloves chopped
- 1 tablespoon salt
- 2 teaspoon paprika
- 1 teaspoon black pepper
- 1 tablespoon cumin
- 1 teaspoon dried oregano
- 2 teaspoons sugar
- 1 teaspoon black pepper

For The Green Sauce

- 3 jalapeno peppers seeded and chopped
- 1 cup cilantro leaves
- 2 cloves garlic chopped
- 1/2 cup mayonnaise
- 1/4 cup sour cream

- 1 tablespoon lime juice
- 1/2 teaspoon salt
- 1/8 teaspoon black pepper
- 2 tablespoon olive oil

Instructions

Blend all the seasoning ingredients for the chicken in the food processor until smooth to make the marinade.

Put the chicken thighs in a large Ziploc bag and pour in the marinade. Marinate the thighs in the refrigerator overnight.

Air fry at 380F (190C) skin side down for about 8-10 minutes. Turn the thighs over and air fry again at 380F (190C) for another 6-8 minutes until temp at 165F (74C).

To make the green sauce, first, blend everything (except olive oil) until smooth. Then, drizzle olive oil slowly and blend to thicken. Refrigerate until ready to serve.

Drizzle the sauce over the chicken or serve it on the side.

Nutrition

Calories:725kcal | Carbohydrates: 9g | Protein: 25g | Fat: 66g | Saturated Fat: 14g | Cholesterol: 161mg

| Sodium: 2343mg | Potassium: 443mg | Fiber: 1g | Sugar: 4g | Vitamin C: 21mg | Calcium: 60mg | Iron: 3mg

Chicken Pasta In Creamy Chimichurri Sauce

Prep Time: 1 hr 30 mins

Cook Time: 15 mins

Ingredients

- 4 pieces of skinless boneless chicken thighs
- 1/4 cup bacon bits
- 2 tbsp butter bacon grease, or olive oil
- 1 tbsp all-purpose flour
- 2/3 cup milk or heavy creamer
- 1 pound cooked spaghetti about 500g or to taste

For The Chimichurri Sauce:

- 1 1/2 cup cilantro minced
- 1/4 cup thinly sliced chives or green onions
- 2 Tablespoon minced garlic
- 2 limes zested and juiced
- 1/2 cup olive oil
- 3 Tablespoon chopped pickled jalapenos
- 1/2 teaspoon sea salt

- 1/4 teaspoon black pepper

Instructions

Use the food processor or a blender to mix all the ingredients for chimichurri sauce for about 10 seconds. Pour about 3/4 cup out and set aside.

In a Ziploc bag, put the chicken pieces in the bag along with the rest of the sauce. Seal the bag, mix, and let them marinate in the refrigerator for at least one hour.

Take the chicken out of the refrigerator 30 minutes before air frying.

Line the fryer basket with a grill mat or a sheet of lightly greased aluminum foil.

Place the chicken inside the fryer basket without stacking. Air fry at 380F (190C) for 10-12 minutes until fully cooked through when the internal temperature exceeds 165F (74C)

In the meantime, heat butter in a wok or a frying pan. Add in flour and stir constantly until it bubbles and thickens. Then, add in milk and 3/4 cup of chimichurri sauce and stir until thickens.

When done, stir in the chicken and serve over pasta. Sprinkle some bacon bits to serve.

Nutrition

Calories:760kcal|Carbohydrates:49g | Protein: 41g | Fat: 45g | Saturated Fat: 10g | Cholesterol: 154mg | Sodium: 829mg | Potassium: 585mg | Fiber: 5g | Sugar: 4g | Vitamin C: 15mg | Calcium: 108mg |Iron: 4mg

Air Fryer Cashew Chicken

Prep Time: 40 mins

Cook Time: 10 mins

Ingredients

- 1 lb boneless and skinless chicken thigh or breast (about 500g) cut into bite-size pieces

Ingredients For Marinade:

- 1/4 cup hoisin sauce
- 1/4 cup soy sauce
- 1 tablespoon white vinegar
- 1 tablespoon sugar
- 2 tablespoon freshly grated ginger
- 1 teaspoon corn starch
- **Other ingredients:**
- 1 teaspoon olive oil
- 2 tablespoon minced garlic
- 1/4 cup steamed carrots diced
- 2 tablespoon scallions
- 1/3 cup roasted cashew halves

Instructions

Mix all the marinade ingredients.

Put the chicken pieces in a Ziploc bag along with 2/3 of the sauce and mix. Marinade the chicken for about 30 minutes. If longer, refrigerate it until cooking.

 Line the fryer basket with a grill mat or a sheet of lightly greased aluminum foil.

Spread the chicken out in the fryer basket and air fry at 380F (190C) for 10-12 minutes until cooked through.

In the meantime, use a wok or a frying pan to saute garlic in olive oil until fragrant, about 1 minute. Add the remaining 1/3 of the marinade and stir constantly until the sauce thickens.

Toss the chicken, carrots, and cashew in the wok to coat. Then, sprinkle some scallions to serve.

Nutrition

Calories: 271kcal | Carbohydrates: 18g | Protein: 29g | Fat: 9g | Saturated Fat: 2g | Cholesterol: 73mg | Sodium: 1228mg | Potassium: 598mg | Fiber: 1g | Sugar: 9g | Vitamin C: 4mg | Calcium: 28mg | Iron: 2mg

Air Fryer Roasted Curry Chicken

Prep Time: 2 hrs

Cook Time: 20 mins

Ingredients

For Chicken:

- 5 pieces skin-on bone-in chicken thighs
- 1/4 cup mayonnaise
- 1 Tablespoon brown sugar
- 1 Tablespoon garlic minced
- 2 Tablespoon soy sauce
- 2 Tablespoon grated ginger
- 1 teaspoon curry powder
- 1/4 teaspoon paprika
- 1/4 teaspoon cumin

Other ingredients:

- 1/2 teaspoon curry powder
- 1/4 teaspoon cumin
- 1/4 teaspoon paprika
- 1/4 cup scallion

Instructions

Mix all the ingredients for chicken. Marinate the chicken in this marinade for at least 2 hours or overnight in the refrigerator.

Mix 1/2 teaspoon of curry, 1/4 teaspoon of cumin, and 1/4 teaspoon of paprika and set aside for later. Take the chicken out of the refrigerator 30 minutes before air frying.

Line the fryer basket with a grill mat or a sheet of lightly greased aluminum foil.

Put the chicken thighs into the basket skin side down, without stacking, and air fry at 380F (190C) for 10 minutes.

Flip the chicken thigh over, now ski side up, and sprinkle some dry seasoning mix over the skin.

Air fry at 380F (190C) for another 6-7 minutes until the meat is cooked through, internal temperature exceeds 170F (77C).

Sprinkle some scallion to serve

Nutrition

Calories: 101kcal | Carbohydrates: 5g | Protein: 1g | Fat: 9g | Saturated Fat: 1g | Cholesterol: 6mg | Sodium: 477mg | Potassium: 41mg | Fiber: 1g | Sugar: 3g | Vitamin C: 1mg | Calcium: 6mg | Iron: 1mg

Yakitori Japanese Skewered Chicken

Prep Time: 1 hr 10 mins

Cook Time: 10 mins

Ingredients

- 1 pound skinless and boneless chicken thigh (about 500g) cut into 1 inch cubes
- 1/4 cup dark soy sauce
- 1/4 cup mirin
- 2 tbsp rice wine
- 2 tbsp brown sugar
- 2 tbsp minced garlic
- 2 tbsp freshly grated ginger
- 1/4 cup scallions for garnish

Instructions

In a large bowl, mix dark soy sauce, mirin, rice wine, brown sugar, garlic, and ginger. Save about 1/3 of the sauce in a small bowl and set aside for later.

Put the chicken thigh cubes in the bowl and mix. Marinate for about 1 hour. Soak the bamboo skewers in water for at least 15 minutes.

Line the fryer basket with a grill mat or a sheet of lightly greased aluminum foil.

Thread the skewers through the chicken pieces then put the skewers in the fryer basket. Spritz some oil over the skewers and air fry at 380F (190C) for 10-12 minutes, flip once in the middle, until the surface is slightly caramelized and the meat is cooked through.

In the meantime, use a saucepan to bring the previously set-aside sauce to boil. Stir constantly until the sauce thickens. Put the sauce in a small bowl to be used for dipping.

Sprinkle the yakitori with scallions and serve with dipping sauce on the side.

Nutrition

Calories:258kcal | Carbohydrates: 28g | Protein: 22g | Fat: 5g | Saturated Fat: 1g | Cholesterol: 108mg | Sodium: 479mg | Potassium: 326mg | Fiber: 1g | Sugar: 20g | Vitamin C: 2mg | Calcium: 27mg | Iron: 1mg

Chicken With Scallion And Ginger Sauce

Prep Time: 5 mins

Marinate At Least One Hour: 20 mins

Ingredients

- 4 pieces of skinless boneless thighs
- 1/2 tsp salt
- 2 tbsp rice wine
- 3 tbsp olive oil
- 1/4 cup dripping from the chicken
- 1/4 cup scallions
- 2 tbsp freshly grated ginger
- 1 tbsp minced garlic
- Salt to taste

Instructions

Marinate the chicken with 1/2 teaspoon of salt and rice wine for at least one hour.

Wrap the thighs in a large, lightly greased aluminum foil (without stacking) and air fry at 380F (190C) for about 15 minutes until the internal temperature exceeds 165F (74C).

When the chicken is done, pour about 1/4 cup of drippings from the foil into a saucepan. Combine it with the rest of the ingredients and bring it to a boil.

Pour the sauce over the chicken to serve.

Nutrition

Calories: 112kcal | Carbohydrates: 2g | Protein: 1g | Fat: 11g | Saturated Fat: 1g | Cholesterol: 1mg | Sodium: 294mg | Potassium: 32mg | Fiber: 1g | Sugar: 1g | Vitamin C: 2mg | Calcium: 8mg | Iron: 1mg

Chicken And Kimchi Fritters

Prep Time: 10 mins

Cook Time: 10 mins

Ingredients

For Chicken:

- 2 cups of chicken fully cooked and shredded
- 1/3 cup kimchi finely shopped
- 1/3 cup Japanese Panko
- 1/4 cup shredded cheese I used Mexican blend
- 2 Tablespoon green onion finely chopped
- 1 Egg beaten

Other ingredients:

- Mayonnaise to taste
- Thinly sliced green onions to taste
- Kimchi to taste

Instructions

Line the fryer basket with a grill mat or a sheet of lightly greased aluminum foil.

Combine all the ingredients. Then, form them into round patties and place them in the fryer basket without stacking.

Air fry at 380F (190C) for about 7-8 minutes, flip once in the middle until the surface is slightly golden brown.

Nutrition

Calories:358kcal | Carbohydrates: 8g | Protein: 28g | Fat: 23g | Saturated Fat: 8g | Cholesterol: 178mg | Sodium: 272mg | Potassium: 264mg | Fiber: 1g | Sugar: 1g | Vitamin C: 3mg | Calcium: 114mg | Iron: 2mg

Thai Chicken Drumsticks

Prep Time: 10 mins

Cook Time: 20 mins

Ingredients For Chicken:

- 8 chicken drumsticks
- 2-3 tablespoon minced garlic
- 3 tablespoon fish sauce
- 2 tablespoon rice wine
- 1 teaspoon sesame oil
- 1 teaspoon black pepper or to taste
- 1/2 teaspoon sriracha hot sauce optional
- 1/4 cup brown sugar
- Juice of one lime

Instructions

Marinate the chicken drumsticks with all the chicken ingredients in a Ziploc bag and refrigerate for at least 3-4 hours, preferably overnight.

Remove the chicken from the refrigerator 30 minutes before air frying.

Line the fryer basket with a grill mat or a sheet of lightly greased aluminum foil.

Air fry at 360F (180C) for about 18-20 minutes until the chicken is cooked through when the internal temperature exceeds 170F (77C).

Drizzle some Thai sweet chili sauce over drumsticks and sprinkle some chopped cilantro to serve.

Nutrition

Calories:324kcal|Carbohydrates:16g | Protein: 28g | Fat: 15g | Saturated Fat: 4g | Cholesterol: 139mg | Sodium: 645mg | Potassium: 411mg | Fiber: 1g | Sugar: 14g | Vitamin C: 2mg | Calcium: 40mg | Iron: 1mg

Curry Chicken Tenderloins

Prep Time: 5 mins

Cook Time: 15 mins

Ingredients

- 4 pieces of chicken tenderloin
- 2 teaspoon coconut oil melted
- 1/2 teaspoon curry powder
- 1/4 teaspoon paprika
- 1/4 teaspoon garlic powder
- 1/4 teaspoon sea salt

Instructions

In a small bowl, mix all the dry ingredients.

Dap dry the tenderloins with a paper towel. Brush coconut oil to both sides of tenderloins. Then, sprinkle the dry ingredients to both sides of the chicken.

Place the tenderloins in the fryer basket. Air fry at 380F (190C) for 10-12 minutes, flip once in the middle until the meat is cooked through when internal temperature exceeds 165F (74C).

Serve the chicken over a bed of greens or rice.

Nutrition

Calories:40kcal | Carbohydrates: 1g | Protein: 3g | Fat: 4g | Saturated Fat: 3g | Cholesterol: 1mg | Sodium: 294mg | Fiber: 1g | Sugar: 1g | Iron: 1mg

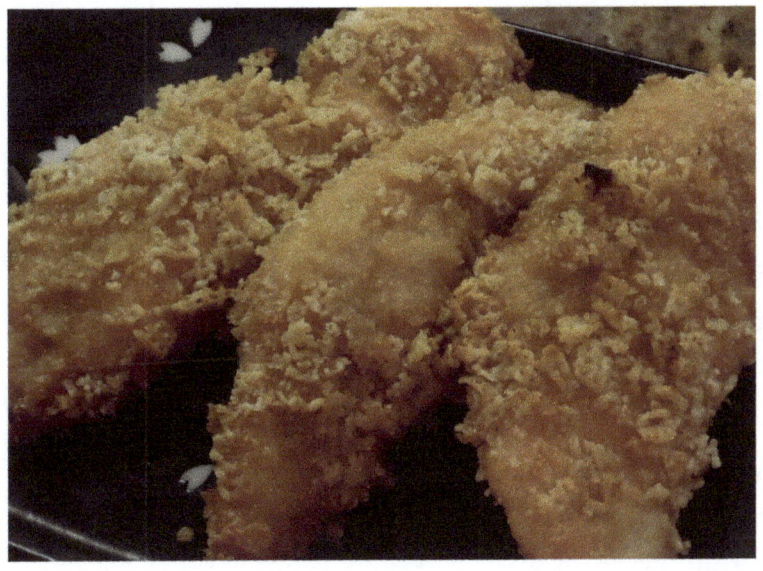

Keto Chicken And Kimchi Rice Bake

Prep Time: 10 mins

Cook Time: 10 mins

Ingredients

- 1 small head of cauliflower
- 2 cups chicken cooked and chopped
- 1 cup kimchi chopped, or to taste
- 2/3 cup juice from kimchi jar or to taste
- 1 cup shredded mozzarella cheese divided, or to taste
- 1 green onion cut into 1/2 inch pieces
- 1/4 cup green onion thinly sliced to garnish (optional)

Instructions

Put the cauliflower into a food processor and pulse it a few times so the cauliflower becomes the size of a grain of rice. Transfer it to a large microwavable bowl and microwave for about 4-5 minutes.

In the meantime, lightly grease a cake pan and set it aside.

When the cauliflower is done, stir in chicken, kimchi, kimchi juice, 2/3 cup of mozzarella cheese, and large green onion pieces. Then, transfer the mixture to the cake pan.

Put the cake pan in the fryer basket and air fry at 360F (180C) for about 4 minutes. Then, sprinkle the rest of the mozzarella cheese over the top and air fry again at 360F (180C) for 3-4 minutes until the cheese melts.

Sprinkle some green onion on to serve.

Nutrition

Calories:181kcal | Carbohydrates: 8g | Protein: 14g | Fat: 11g | Saturated Fat: 5g | Cholesterol: 42mg | Sodium: 239mg | Potassium: 520mg | Fiber: 3g | Sugar: 3g | Vitamin C: 71mg | Calcium: 181mg | Iron: 1mg

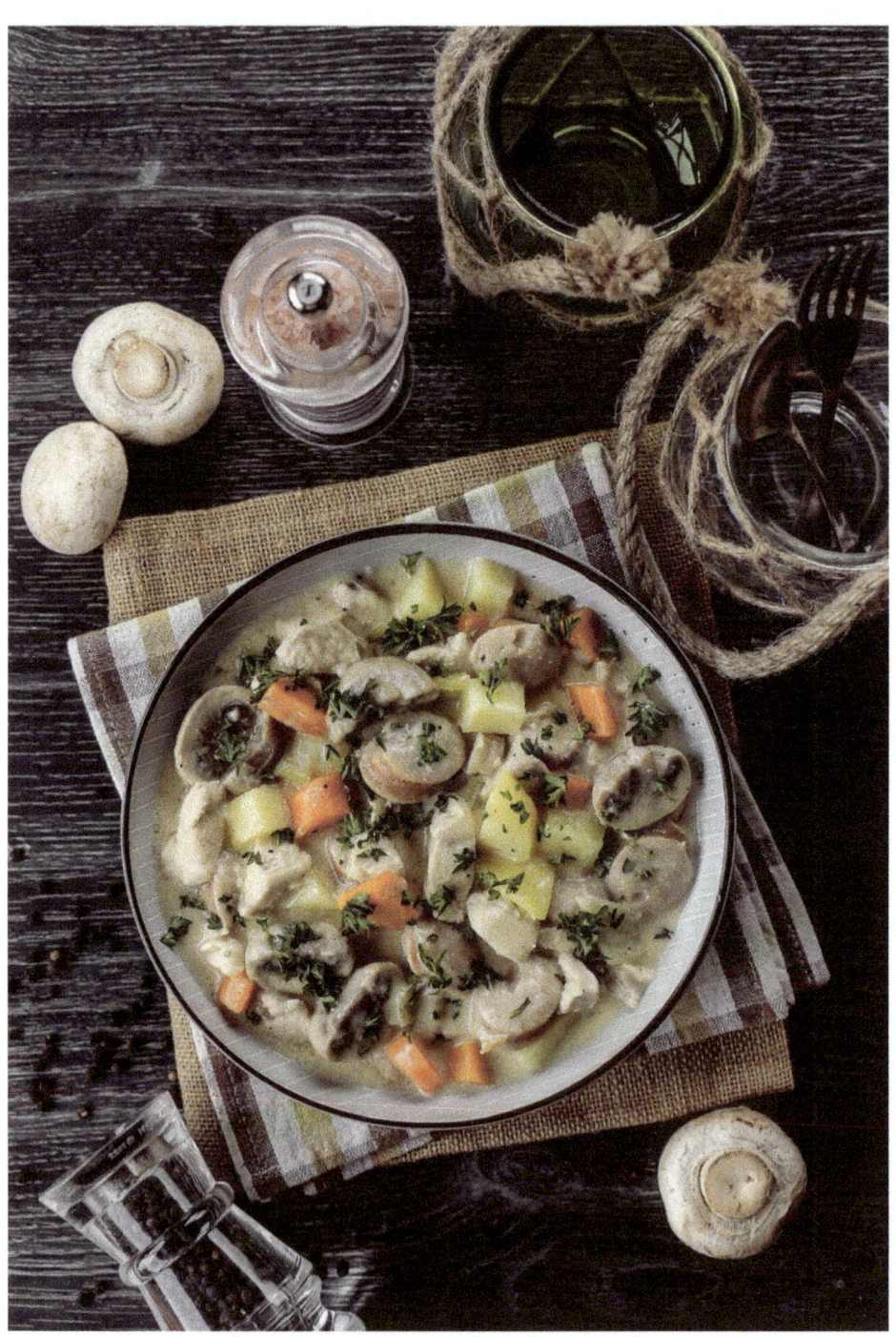

Lightning Source UK Ltd.
Milton Keynes UK
UKHW020652300421
382894UK00005B/40